Adrenal Fatigue

*How to Reduce Stress,
Boost Your Energy Levels,
and Overcome Adrenal
Burnout Using the
Adrenal Reset Diet*

By
Jacob Wilson

Table of Contents

Introduction.

Adrenal Fatigue - An Overview

Even though adrenal fatigue was first given this name by Dr. James Wilson back in 1998, this term is not new. This is actually a syndrome with a lot of names, for instance, it has been called non-Addisonís hypoadrenia; chronic fatigue syndrome; neurasthenia; sub-clinical hypoadrenia, adrenal neurasthenia; adrenal apathy and adrenal disorder. Medically it is officially called hypoadrenia.

Regardless of what it's called, this syndrome is recognized by tiredness, problems with digestive system, difficulty sleeping, aches and nervousness. Many different symptoms could be related to adrenal fatigue, which makes it a syndrome instead of a disease. It's a name directed at a group of non-specific symptoms.

All of these symptoms can be related to a problem with the adrenal glands. For instance, stress will cause the adrenal glands to make specific hormones such as cortisol. In case stress continues over a prolonged time period, the adrenal glands might be incapable of producing the same level of hormones. This would mean that the hormones that body needs will not be supplied so you will experience adrenal fatigue symptoms. This syndrome can be brought on by any form of stress, whether it's mental, physical, spiritual or emotional.

As expected the primary symptom that individuals with this syndrome will experience would be fatigue. However, this fatigue isn't the usual tiredness that disappears after a day off from work, vacation or even a good night sleep. The truth is those who have this syndrome generally feel exhausted most of the time, especially in the mornings. They might depend on stimulants including coffee and cola to get through the entire day. For severe cases, these people might get up for a couple of hours and then return to bed.

In most cases, adrenal fatigue might be a contributing factor for many different conditions, which include obesity and allergies. Although doctors generally check the adrenal glands using blood tests, those tests can be notoriously incorrect in revealing the concentrations of adrenal hormones such as cortisol, testosterone, adrenaline, and estrogen. Blood tests are basically not sensitive enough to identify the small reductions in adrenal function which might be triggering this problem.

Addisonís disease, which is the polar extreme of hypoadrenia, also shares a few of the symptoms such as fatigue and body aches. Addisonís disease could also lead to weight loss, low blood pressure, lightheadedness and loss of body hair. This will be due to an adrenal insufficiency, which is the insufficient creation of hormones by the adrenal glands. Blood tests and various other medical checkups could be used to confirm the diagnosis of this disease.

What Is Adrenal Fatigue?

What exactly is 'adrenal fatigue'? According to proponents, it is a maladaptive state in which adrenal hormone production is significantly decreased in response to repeated and chronic psychological stress; the resulting state of 'hypoadrenia' then renders the body incapable of perpetuating an adaptive constant fight or flight response or mounting an appropriate stress response to acute stressors. As one major advocate of the term states, "The adrenals simply cannot keep up with demands placed upon them." So, if adrenal fatigue is not accurate or useful, what do healthcare providers, whether conventional or alternative, have to gain from applying and promoting this diagnosis? The reasons vary and include everything from misunderstanding and misinformation to personal financial gain.

What are adrenal glands and whats makes them so important?

About the size of a thumb, adrenal glands sit at top your kidneys and produce hormones that help you deal with stress. These two little organs are responsible for our bodies response to stress and lets us cope with it. They produce, release and regulate hormones such as cortisol and adrenaline that are responsible for our moods. That is why cortisol is also known as "stress hormone". Adrenal glands also produces hormone known as DHEA (an anabolic or building hormone). DHEA hormone is our body's natural anti-inflammatory and an aldosterone which balances minerals in in our body.

Under normal circumstances, adrenal glands secrete small amounts of these regulatory substances. But when you are in danger, either real or perceived, they flood your body with adrenal hormones, particularly norepinephrine (adrenaline) and cortisol, that activate the fight-or-flight response. The purpose of this response is to prepare your body for battle by giving you greater strength, mental clarity, and energy.

Because stress is a fact of modern life, most us have norepinephrine and cortisol coursing through our bodies when we are in no real danger. As a result, our adrenal glands have to work overtime to keep up with the more or less constant demand. It is not surprising then that our adrenals can occasionally become overdrawn, forcing the body to deal with stress at a hormonal deficit. This condition is known as adrenal fatigue.

While the adrenal glands do play a definite role in how we feel day to day (whether that's energetic or exhausted), as we've now established, the term "adrenal fatigue" is, at best, a misnomer. According to several medical establishments in disagreement with this concept, the term adrenal fatigue is used by some doctors of alternative medicine who claim adrenal fatigue to be too mild to be picked up on standard blood tests. Research goes on to state that proponents of this "unproven term claim it to be a mild form of adrenal insufficiency rendering a patient incapable of producing enough stress hormones to produce an adequate fight or flight response."

Medical research on Adrenal Fatigue.

Is adrenal fatigue real or imagined.

Although modern doctors are more open-minded about unknown or unclassified illnesses than they were in the past, many patients still face skepticism when they complain about conditions that do not fit neatly into any accepted category. In these instances, doctors sometimes surmise that the symptoms are influenced by the patient's mental or emotional state. Such is the case with adrenal fatigue, a syndrome that has grown increasingly common in the U.S.

Even though there are similar disorders that affect the adrenal glands in similar ways, adrenal fatigue is not an accepted medical condition. There are a lot of reasons for this, most of which concern the different ways human beings process and handle stress. For example, we know that tests can measure cortisol levels in the blood as well as the saliva. They can even tell doctors if the adrenal glands are producing enough hormones to deal with daily stress. However, there are no clear facts among medical professionals about what constitutes low levels on these tests. Doctors also know that people have different numbers of cortisol receptors that help determine how well adrenal hormones work to reduce anxiety and stress. In fact, most researchers believe that adrenal fatigue is caused, at least in part, by the interactions between the adrenal glands and the brain.

We may all agree that adrenal fatigue is caused by chronic stress. We do not know why it affects some people and not others or how it can be effectively treated on a long-term basis. Then again, it was only recently that disturbances in the central nervous system and neurotransmitters were identified by science and accepted by the medical establishment. In other words, we have much to learn before the condition is understood and accepted.

If we look to the roots from whence this mammoth tree emerges, we will find them grounded in the desperation of millions of chronically stressed, depressed, and fatigued people for whom conventional medicine has no answer. The level of frustration is high all the time, and patients often leave the office of their healthcare provider in despair when they are told that all of their test results are 'in the normal range' and that an anti-depressant prescription is in order.

.

Recent findings.

Although the link between depression and adrenal fatigue requires additional investigation, researchers have established that it does indeed exist. In one recent study, the mean adrenal gland volume was 70 percent higher while patients were depressed than it was after they were successfully treated for their illness. While testing for adrenal fatigue was not completed in that study, it stands to reason that adrenals that were working 70 percent harder to pump out stress hormones would be more likely to suffer from fatigue than those that were operating normally. It is not a large leap then to deduce that chronic stress can cause depression and later adrenal fatigue, which can wreak havoc on your life.

Medical Research Confirms The Existence Adrenal Fatigue.

Many years of research on adrenal fatigue have provided clear-cut evidence that low cortisol states do exist and contribute to disease formation. In fact, up to 25% of all stress-related human disorders (PTSD, chronic fatigue syndrome, fibromyalgia, irritable bowel syndrome, etc.) are associated with low cortisol states. However, the medical terminology used to describe low cortisol has everything to do with acceptance of, proper diagnosis of, and evidence-based treatment for this condition. Patients shun from uttering the words 'adrenal fatigue' to their doctor for fear of being chastised and ignored, and I am speaking from direct personal experience. The medically appropriate term for low cortisol states is known as hypocortisolism, and it is true that conventional medical testing often misses the diagnosis. This is where the dichotomy between conventional 'black and white' and more integrative 'shades of gray' diverge.

Convergence of these diametrically opposed medical factions is evolving and ultimately inevitable. In the interim, the millions of people suffering from symptoms of hypocortisolism will remain undiagnosed at the hands of their conventional medical doctors and therefore self-treat as they continue to seek medical advice and purchase the nutritional supplements from the internet based 'adrenal fatigue' gurus, many of whom lack MD degrees. Buyers beware!

Causes of Adrenal Fatigue

There are many possible causes of fatigue, but the most common include overwork, poor diet, and subclinical hormone imbalances (of the endocrine system). Unfortunately, many of these problems are under-diagnosed as blood tests only identify severe cases.

Most common cause of adrenal fatigue is adrenal hormone deficiency.

Let's start with the basics. Think of the adrenal glands as the body's master stress gland. The adrenals produce cortisol (commonly known as the stress hormone) and many other hormones to help the body go into overdrive mode during times of high stress. This is sustainable for shorter periods of time, but prolonged elevated stress levels tax the body's adrenal glands and do not allow for rest and recovery.

Many kinds of stress can tax the adrenal glands: chemical stress, thermal stress, physical stress, and mental/emotional stress. Chemical stress can come from a diet low in necessary nutrients or from a diet too high in sugar and processed foods. Environmental exposure to toxins and chemicals also increases the amount of chemical stress. Rapid changes in temperature and barometric pressure place extra thermal stress on the body. Overworking, over-training, and lack of sleep are all examples of physical stressors. And mental/emotional stressors range from financial insecurity to fighting to grief over the loss of a loved one.

Some people have stronger constitutions (more active adrenal glands) and can seemingly handle more stress than others, however, no one is immune to the effects of stress. It is a mistake to expect our bodies to run at a superhuman pace for extended periods of time.

Signs And Symptoms of Adrenal Fatigue.

Adrenal fatigue usually comes in different signs and symptoms to various people. Its variation often leads some to think that there is actually nothing wrong with the extreme feelings of tiredness that they are experiencing since people believe that being tired is actually normal for human beings.

Truthfully, people get tired after doing hard work and hours of labor, but the thing is that people are also able to generally cope with the exhaustion. When people do things that they normally can't do they get stressed and when they continue doing so even after that their body has already signaled fatigue then that is where adrenal fatigue comes in.

Adrenal fatigue is a form of stress that lasts for a very long time unless attended with the utmost care. When not treated appropriately, adrenal fatigue might lead to depression and also causes the body's immune system to decrease thus increasing the risk of having infections and other forms of diseases

While adrenal fatigue is not yet recognized as a legitimate disorder, adrenal insufficiency (Addison's disease) is. However, the main difference between the 2 is that adrenal insufficiency results in either complete adrenal failure or extremely low adrenal function called hypoadrenia. Adrenal fatigue is actually caused by the different disorder, hyperadrenia, which is an over activity of the adrenal glands due to increased need. With that said, the two diseases result in similar complications in patients.

As we know, the adrenal glands help us manage stress. They were not, however, designed to deal with prolonged periods of anxiety that last for days, weeks, even months on end. These major depressive episodes not only result in elevated stress levels, but they may also be exacerbated by the continued release of cortisol and other stress hormones in response to the symptoms of depression, such as fatigue, poor sleep, anxiety, and mental exhaustion.

Common signs of adrenal fatigue that should help you distinguish it from normal fatigue:

- Always tired. The thing that separates adrenal or severe chronic fatigue from the normal fatigue is that the exhaustion that an individual feel when having adrenal fatigue lasts for weeks, months and even years. The energy just drops to the point wherein you find it very hard to wake up and perform even the simplest tasks and daily duties.

- Decreased libido. People who are under mild stress generally find sex as a stress reliever. But with people having adrenal or severe chronic fatigue, it seems that their sex drive is too low that they don't have the energy and the passion for performing sexually.
- Decreased immunity. People who are stressed don't typically develop reduced immunity but with people having adrenal or severe chronic fatigue, their immune system drops thus making them prone to infections such as cold and flu.
- Reduced focus. If you've noticed before, mild stress can actually help you perform better at work, at home, and at school. But with people having adrenal or severe chronic fatigue, the stress they experience is too much that it often leads to anxiety and panic attacks.

Other symptoms of adrenal fatigue include:

- dizziness when first standing up
- excess inflammation and pain (this includes arthritis, tendonitis, dermatitis, and more
- trouble sleeping

It's tempting to believe that the way out of the tired mess we've gotten our bodies into is an energy drink or a cup of coffee, but this is not a long-term solution. These drinks force the already tired adrenal glands to work harder. This is analogous to kicking a horse when it's exhausted to get it to work some more. Abuse of caffeine and energy drinks (with high doses of synthetic B vitamins) has a very real toll on our bodies.

These are only a few of the common signs of adrenal fatigue. If you're experiencing the above mentioned for several weeks of months now, then you should be warned and start with your recovery action now before it's actually too late!

General disinterest. Stress does not usually affect your vigor with life, but people who experience adrenal or severe chronic fatigue usually end up losing interest in things they usually love like work, hobbies and much more.

Three stages of Adrenal Fatigue

During the 1950s a famous researcher called Hans Seyle wanted to know what happens to animals under stress. It turned out that when stressed, both rats and people react in similar ways.

She found out that there was a large quantity of Cortisol were produced when one is stressed, the level of cortisol decreases when fear fades away. Many people actually enjoy this initial feeling when there is the high production of cortisol (high-cortisol rush). High cortisol levels in the body is very essential to keep our spirits high when we need to be, but when our bodies stay in this state for long, things will start falling apart. This initial stage where there is a huge rush of cortisol is called stage one.

Continued production of high cortisol may render adrenal glands to burn out due to the high stress put on them, their ability to keep producing cortisol starts to decline. Stage two begins when cortisol level drops out and depletes.

Stage Three is reached when the cortisol level has fallen to extremely low concentrations, and its production depletes, and the body starts to shut down. In this stage, you will experience some symptoms and illness.

When the adrenal glands weaken, cortisol production drops immensely, the body ends up storing a lot of body fat around the abdominals around your belly, the energy levels also drop and you start experiencing fatigue all the time, and bad moods set in because your cortisol levels have been depressed. Finally, some people start developing heartburn, ulcers, and other digestive problems. Burn out of cortisol concentrations in both women and men can be severe, as sex hormones may burn out leading to erectile dysfunction in men and hormone imbalances in women. High cortisol levels have many disadvantages. It destroys the cardiovascular function and the heart, and freezes the brain, triggering memory loss and depresses thyroid function. Thousands of research done over the years have shown that low levels of cortisol have translated to long term degenerative diseases including diabetes, heart disease and even cancer.

Stage 1: Stress

Whatever the source of stress, whether its physical, emotional, inflammation, chemical, infection or trauma, the body's initial reaction will remain the same i.e. the adrenal glands produce more stress hormones, cortisol, and adrenaline. At this stage, you are able to burn the candle at both ends. You can wake up very early and sleep up very late, or even pull a 24 hour without sleep and still recover quickly just on the next sleep This first stage of hormonal maladaptation is known as hyperadrenia, or over activity of adrenal glands. In a typical reaction to stress, when stress level decreases, adrenal glands have time to recondition and be prepared for the next event of pressure. However, if the stress level continues and remains high, the body will burn out and remain locked. If the degree of stress hormone remains high for long periods, the body's ability to recover fully becomes a problem and the ability of adrenals to produce cortisol and DHEA will be compromised.

Elevated levels of cortisol have a significant effect on the brain. It damages the cells in your hippocampus, this is the part of the brain responsible for learning and memory, which leads to poor memory. When both adrenaline and cortisol levels are both high, it puts your mind in in an extremely high state of alertness, ready to do anything, ready to run or fight.

You will know if you are experiencing stage one of Adrenal Fatigue if you:

- Have trouble on falling asleep or staying asleep.
- Feel your hormones are out of whack.
- Gaining weight and increased abdominal fat.

- Going through blood sugar fluctuations.
- May feel very exhausted even after more eight hours of sleep.

Stage 2: Fatigue

Some people have genetically strong glands and can handle stress and maintain good health under high levels of stress for a long time. But if the individual does not make the necessary dietary and lifestyle changes, prolonged stress will eventually enter into stage 2 of adrenal fatigue. This transition period usually lasts between 6-18 months, gradually adrenal glands can't handle such a depression and gets compromised.

Most people will notice their ability to carry out their daily duties and tasks plunges, and they can't do a lot of work like before. But their levels of consuming stimulants increase such as caffeine or self-medicated supplements. In this stage of adrenal maladaptation, most individuals will realize that something is not the same, and their resistance to high levels of stress is decreasing. Organs, tissues, and cells in the body begin to function abnormally because they are adapting to stress poorly.

Besides recognizing the energy fall off, people in this stage may start experiencing low thyroid function, salt and sugar cravings and detoxification problems. Skin disorders, psoriasis, rashes, eczema and other skin problems may also appear. Decreased sex drive. Back pain, neck and other muscle related pains and aches begin. Allergies, infections, and sensitiveness food surface or worsen. Standard medical testing may show that everything is normal, and the doctor may recommend medication for symptomatic relief.

Under chronic stress, adrenals burn out gradually or quickly. At this stage, the glands become completely fatigued and can no longer handle an adequate response to stress. This condition ultimately leads to the final stage of adrenal fatigue.

Stage 3: Exhaustion.

This is the final stage, also known as hypoadrenalism. In this juncture of adrenal maladaptation, the glands burn out and of their ability to make cortisol and DHEA in adequate amounts is depleted. Therefore it becomes more and more difficult for the body to recover as days goes by. Low-level depression and constant fatigue may also appear in emotionally healthy people and stress-free individuals because the DHEA and cortisol help maintain energy levels, keep moods and stabilize emotions.

When cortisol and DHEA levels in the body are insufficient, individuals experience depressed mental function. Brain activity suffers as these hormones are inadequate. Both mental confusion and poor memory can be a direct result of adrenal hormone depletion. This is now when some people seek medical attention for symptoms and/or pain related disorders. Blood sugar worsens, and muscle mass begins to decrease. Individuals in this stage become sick more often, and they do not recover like they used to. The person usually finds it difficult to wake up in the morning and feels tired throughout the day. Stimulants such as caffeine that helped in the past is not working like before, and the need for stimulants is intensifying.

Stage three patients are often worn out and exhausted. They just can't regain their strength back no matter what they do or many visits they make to the doctor. In this stage diseases are diagnosable, and symptom relief is often prescribed, neglecting the primary cause.

Getting Tested for Adrenal Fatigue.

Medical tests on adrenal fatigue.

With the demands of today's hectic work schedules, feeling fatigued is an all-too-common occurrence. Feeling this way once in a while for short periods of time is not cause for concern, but persistent fatigue may be an indicator that there is something wrong. Symptoms that may warrant an examination include:

- Feeling a dramatic slump in energy after lunchtime
- Consistent difficulty waking up in the morning
- Constant reliance on "pick-me-ups" such as caffeine, sugar, or energy drinks
- Feeling demotivated and lacking energy for essential daily activities

It is important for anyone to determine whether they are experiencing Adrenal fatigue. This is because it takes physical symptoms like the ones mentioned before a person will even want to investigate what could be wrong with them, getting the adrenal hormone levels tested is the primary indication to detect any sign of adrenal fatigue.

There are two hormones mostly tested to determine if a person is suffering from adrenal fatigue. These hormones, cortisol, and DHEA are the best indicators of how well the adrenal glands are functioning. You can even test for adrenal fatigue from home using home "saliva tests" to check these hormones. These saliva test kits are relatively inexpensive and are available online through some companies and are also available in many pharmacies

Saliva testing of adrenal hormones is known for being reliable and accurate. It is recognized by medical research groups, including the U.S National Institutes of Health – National Library of Medicine (PubMed). If adrenal hormones are found to be insufficient even if it is slightly below the normal range, this is a more definite sign of adrenal fatigue.

To be evaluated for a subclinical adrenal condition, see a natural medicine practitioner who is familiar with salivary hormone testing (the Adrenal Stress Index by DiagnosTechs), the Koenisburg test, and Professional Applied Kinesiology (PAK). PAK involves neurological testing of muscles and reflexes; as there are certain specific muscles in the body whose dysfunction has been clinically correlated with adrenal dysfunction, this is a great tool to help in the identification and treatment of adrenal insufficiency. Treatment may include supplements specially formulated to aid in adrenal recovery.

Many doctors do not recognize adrenal fatigue but will only detect the severe type of adrenal hypofunction, called Addison's disease. Due to this Doctors believe that a person who passes a test called the ATCH Stimulation Test, which is designed to detect a full blown adrenal insufficiency, needs no further tests. This mild adrenal fatigue may develop into severe symptoms. A person with adrenal fatigue will pass this test, in most cases. Therefore, the best approach is to check the levels of the main adrenal hormones, Cortisol and DHEA.

The ACTH Stimulation Test is designed to test the adrenal reaction which is stimulated by Pituitary hormone ACTH. The problem with this analysis is that with adrenal fatigue, the adrenal glands can be stimulated and will react but may still produce low levels of adrenal hormones which usually end up crushing afterward due to extra stimulation because of small adrenal reserves.

Adrenals play a significant role in our immune system. When adrenals aren't functioning well, this may cause some serious issues such as allergy, viral and illness responses to occur. Cortisol hormone also plays a significant role in our body's natural anti-inflammatory defense. Low levels of Cortisol in our body gives rise to muscle and joint pains and other inflammatory reactions in the body. When all these mild issues are combined, they contribute to the symptoms of adrenal fatigue. These symptoms can add struggles to patients with hypothyroid who have these co-morbid conditions.

In fact, adrenal fatigue can be a major contributing factor to these and other chronic syndromes and diseases or may also not be related to any particular condition at all.

It is, therefore, crucial when one feel that they may have adrenal fatigue to be tested immediately because other hormone deficiency and imbalances can cause similar responses. A lot of pharmacies have the "ZRT Labs" saliva hormone kits, including the ones that test levels adrenal and sex hormone as well.

Three Self Tests you can do by yourself at home.

Well, how do you know if you are among the 80% who have adrenal fatigue? Well, you may examine your lifestyle at home by just performing some straightforward and easy tests to tell whether you are suffering from adrenal fatigue. Additionally, if you seem not to catch up on your sleep, or you are chronically tired and grumpy, you are likely to be suffering from this problem. Here are three simple adrenal fatigue tests you can administer to see if your adrenal glands are functioning well or they need help.

Pupil Dilation

In this test, you need a mirror and a flashlight. Then look into the mirror and shine the flashlight into the pupil of one of your eye. The pupil should contract pretty quickly. If your pupil does not contract after 30 seconds, or even dilates, then your adrenals need some help.

Ragland's Test

This test involves checking of blood pressure and therefore you will need a home blood pressure machine (you can buy one for around $10 at any drug store). First, when sitting down take a blood pressure, then stand up and record your blood pressure again, right away. Your systolic number (the first or top number) should increase by 8 or 10 points. If the number drops, then you probably have adrenal fatigue

Pain and Sensitivity

Adrenal glands are located right on top of kidneys. If you palpate that area and feel pain, then your adrenal glands are fatigued. You can also try pressing on the reflexology point for the adrenal glands, which is located at the top inside edge of your foot arch. If that area is sensitive, then so are your adrenal glands.

Treatment of Adrenal Fatigue.

In more severe cases, patients with adrenal fatigue have a hard time waking up and getting out of bed. They may sleep and sleep and sleep, but since the problem is in their adrenal glands, slumber will not restore their diminished energy levels. And since adrenal hormones have a profound effect on cognitive function, mood, and mental states, they may find it difficult to escape anxiety and depression.

Even if they do not accept adrenal fatigue as the likely cause of a possible illness, doctors can complete tests that measure the hormonal output of the adrenal glands. But since they fluctuate wildly throughout the day, it is important to get multiple types of blood and/or saliva tests to establish a baseline for cortisol levels. It is also crucial for patients to try to limit stress while they take these tests since increases in anxiety will result in false positives and negatives from cortisol levels. If you are diagnosed and you find out that you are suffering from adrenal insufficiency, there is a lot of ways to get it treated.

Antidepressants

Because they know that stress forces the adrenal glands into overdrive and that the hormones they release can cause depression, doctors almost always turn to antidepressants to treat the symptoms of the underlying problem. Of course, that will not solve the problem, i.e., that the adrenal glands are not working as they should. This is the primary reason that many patients have turned to alternative medicine to treat this modern malady.

Adaptogens

When adrenal glands can't meet the demand of daily stress, you undergo you will likely develop an adrenal fatigue. Research has shown that people suffering from adrenal fatigue have nothing wrong with their glands, but rather with the amount of stress the person encounters on a daily basis. Therefore, the only way to treat adrenal fatigue is to find healthy, productive ways to cope with stress. Our prescription? Eat right, exercise, get a good nights' sleep, and take dietary supplements.

One group of supplements that may help reduce stress and support healthy adrenal function at the same time is adaptogens. These safe and effective herbal medicines have been used in both Hindu and Chinese traditional medicines to ease stress and anxiety for thousands of years. Natural supplements with no known drug interactions, adaptogens such as ashwagandha, ginseng, maca, licorice root, and Rhodiola are available for sale on the internet. When using adaptogens to treat adrenal fatigue, be sure to follow the recommended dosage.

Natural ways to treat adrenal fatigue.

Although the quick fix is tempting, the only real, natural, and non-toxic solutions are the following measures:

1. Get at least 7 to 9 hours of sleep per night.
2. Allow yourself some time for rest each week.
3. Do not skip meals; low blood sugar levels place extra stress on the adrenals.
4. Do not eat sugary, high-carb foods; this causes a blood sugar crash afterward, known as the "carb stupor."
5. Exercise only aerobically until you've recovered to avoid further fatigue and further stress to the adrenal glands. Get a heart rate monitor and follow this formula to calculate your proper heart rate zone: maximum heart rate is 180 minus your current age; subtract another 10 for your minimum heart rate.
6. Get evaluated for a hormone imbalance by a doctor trained in Applied Kinesiology to determine which supplements and what therapies (chiropractic, homeopathy, or acupuncture) can help restore adrenal health as quickly as possible.

If you are diagnosed with adrenal insufficiency, a combination of some or all of the above measures is optimal. It usually takes adrenal glands two to three months for them to fully recover, but the lasting, long-term improvement in energy and health are well worth the effort.

Can Supplements Really Help with Adrenal Fatigue?

Adrenal fatigue is experienced by a large segment of the population, estimated at approximately 80% of people in industrialized countries. Many people have discovered that supplements can help rebuild worn out adrenal glands.

While it is true that doctors have shown that adrenal glands can indeed return to full health through supplementation, it is generally not your first step when implementing a treatment plan.

When considering, adrenal supplements keep in mind that adrenal fatigue is more often than not caused by neglecting health and stress recovery. Often it is due primarily to poor lifestyle and a diet filled with sugar, fats, caffeine, and other stimulants. This is further complicated in that most of us don't receive enough nutrients or vitamins. This explains why our adrenal glands give out, and we begin feeling extreme tiredness no matter what we do.

Your treatments will vary depending on the severity of your symptoms. Although supplements will absolutely be a part of your treatment, other plans to help you better deal with stress and get proper nutrition will also need to be put in place.

Supplements help by giving your adrenal glands and the rest of your cells the building material they require to replenish waning supplies of nutrients. Adrenal glandular in particular will be helpful in the actual rebuilding of the adrenal glands. When considering treatment for a full recovery from adrenal fatigue, supplements are vital.

You will want to alter your diet as well. Concentrate on getting enough protein, complex carbs, and vitamin c, b, and d. The foods to avoid are those that are high in fat and sugar. Eat plenty of vegetables, but make sure to get them in different varieties and colors. Make sure to eat them (as well as all foods) as close to their original state as possible as much of the nutritional value will be lost through age, processing, canning, freezing, and cooking. Also drink water instead of alcohol, caffeine, soda, or sugar filled drinks.

Conclusion.

The debate over whether or not adrenal fatigue is an actual disease is unlikely to end anytime soon. However, we can all agree that rising levels of stress and strain have very real, often deleterious effects on our health. The link between depression and chronic stress is now accepted by members of the medical community. Adrenal fatigue is precipitated by these prolonged bouts of anxiety and depression that force the adrenal glands into overdrive and gradually wear them down. Those that suffer from this increasingly common disorder must find healthy and effective treatment options, such as adaptogens, to help them manage daily stress.